This journa

Name: _____

Mobile: _____

E-mail: _____

Age: _____

Weight: _____

Height: _____

Paleo Diet

You've accepted the challenge - Yay! Welcome to 30 Days of Paleo! Here's a way to keep track of your diet. Don't forget that there's a Paleo Journal to help you! which is easily sortable with Nutrition info & Net/Total Carb Counts. You can do it! GOOD LUCK

STARTING WEIGHT: **Day30 WEIGHT:**

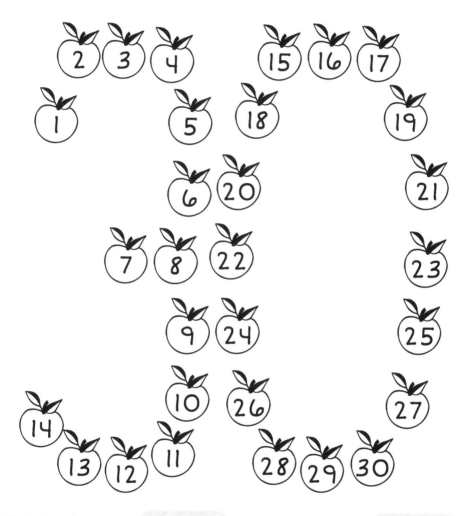

Total weight lost: Total inches lost:

CONGRATS! YOU DID THAT ! YOU MADE IT!
NOW LET'S DO ANOTHER ROUND OF 60 DAYS OF PALEO!

FIRST OF BODY MEASUREMENTS

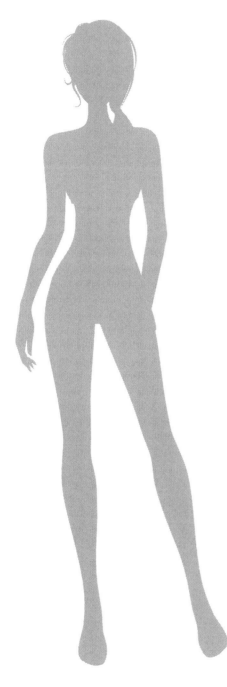

NECK:

Left Arm:

Right Arm:

CHEST:

WAIST:

HIPS:

Left Thigh:

Right Thigh:

Left Calf:

Right Calf:

Weight:

Heart Rate:

Blood Pressure:

END OF MEASUREMENTS

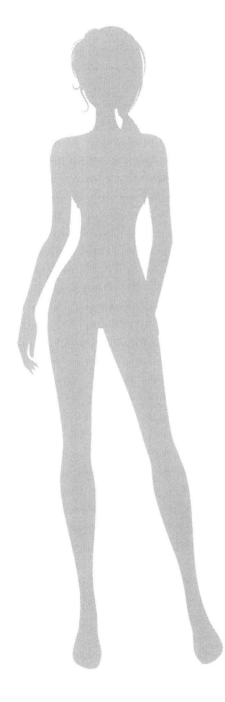

NECK:

Left Arm:

Right Arm:

CHEST:

WAIST:

HIPS:

Left Thigh:

Right Thigh:

Left Calf:

Right Calf:

Weight:

Heart Rate:

Blood Pressure:

Wake Time

Paleo Food Log

Day 1

Sleep Time

DATE:

JAN FEB MAR APR MAY JUN JUL AUG SEP OCT NOV DEC

Breakfast:

Calories: _____

Lunch:

Calories: _____

Dinner:

Calories: _____

Snack:

Calories: _____

Water Intake

☐ Vegetables&Fruits
☐ Meats&Seafood
☐ Eggs, Nuts& Seeds
☐ Healthy Oils

Vitamins [_____]   Medicine [_____]

🏋 Today's Workout	CALORIES	WEIGHT

Today I feel.....

NOTES

_____
_____
_____
_____

Wake Time

Sleep Time

Paleo Food Log

Day 2

DATE:

Breakfast:

Calories:

Lunch:

Calories:

Dinner:

Calories:

Snack:

Calories:

Water Intake

Vitamins

Medicine

- [ ] Vegetables&Fruits
- [ ] Meats&Seafood
- [ ] Eggs, Nuts& Seeds
- [ ] Healthy Oils

Today's Workout	CALORIES	WEIGHT

Today I feel.....

NOTES

Wake Time

Sleep Time

Paleo Food Log

DATE:

JAN FEB MAR APR MAY JUN JUL AUG SEP OCT NOV DEC

Breakfast:

Calories: _____

Lunch:

Calories: _____

Dinner:

Calories: _____

Snack:

Calories: _____

Water Intake

☐ **Vegetables&Fruits**
☐ **Meats&Seafood**
☐ **Eggs, Nuts& Seeds**
☐ **Healthy Oils**

Vitamins _____ **Medicine** _____

🏋 Today's Workout	CALORIES	WEIGHT

Today I feel.....

NOTES

_____
_____
_____
_____

Wake Time

Sleep Time

Paleo Food Log

DATE:

JAN FEB MAR APR MAY JUN JUL AUG SEP OCT NOV DEC

Breakfast:

Calories:

Lunch:

Calories:

Dinner:

Calories:

Snack:

Calories:

Water Intake

Vitamins

Medicine

- [ ] Vegetables&Fruits
- [ ] Meats&Seafood
- [ ] Eggs, Nuts& Seeds
- [ ] Healthy Oils

Today's Workout	CALORIES	WEIGHT

Today I feel.....

NOTES

Wake Time

Sleep Time

Paleo Food Log

Day
5

DATE:

JAN FEB MAR APR MAY JUN JUL AUG SEP OCT NOV DEC

Breakfast:

Calories:

Lunch:

Calories:

Dinner:

Calories:

Snack:

Calories:

Water Intake

- [ ] Vegetables&Fruits
- [ ] Meats&Seafood
- [ ] Eggs, Nuts& Seeds
- [ ] Healthy Oils

Vitamins

Medicine

Today's Workout	CALORIES	WEIGHT

Today I feel.....

NOTES

Wake Time

Sleep Time

Paleo Food Log

| Day 6 |

DATE:

JAN FEB MAR APR MAY JUN JUL AUG SEP OCT NOV DEC

Breakfast:

Calories: _____

Lunch:

Calories: _____

Dinner:

Calories: _____

Snack:

Calories: _____

Water Intake

⬜ **Vegetables&Fruits**
⬜ **Meats&Seafood**
⬜ **Eggs, Nuts& Seeds**
⬜ **Healthy Oils**

Vitamins _____   **Medicine** _____

Today's Workout	CALORIES	WEIGHT

Today I feel.....

NOTES

Wake Time

Sleep Time

Paleo Food Log

Day
7

DATE:

JAN FEB MAR APR MAY JUN JUL AUG SEP OCT NOV DEC

Breakfast:

Calories:

Lunch:

Calories:

Dinner:

Calories:

Snack:

Calories:

Water Intake

Vitamins

Medicine

- [ ] **Vegetables&Fruits**
- [ ] **Meats&Seafood**
- [ ] **Eggs, Nuts& Seeds**
- [ ] **Healthy Oils**

Today's Workout	CALORIES	WEIGHT

Today I feel.....

NOTES

Wake Time

Sleep Time

Paleo Food Log

Day 8

DATE:

JAN FEB MAR APR MAY JUN JUL AUG SEP OCT NOV DEC

Breakfast:

Calories:

Lunch:

Calories:

Dinner:

Calories:

Snack:

Calories:

Water Intake

☐ Vegetables&Fruits
☐ Meats&Seafood
☐ Eggs, Nuts& Seeds
☐ Healthy Oils

Vitamins [   ]   Medicine [   ]

🏋 Today's Workout	CALORIES	WEIGHT

Today I feel.....

NOTES

Wake Time

Sleep Time

Paleo Food Log

Day 9

DATE:

JAN FEB MAR APR MAY JUN JUL AUG SEP OCT NOV DEC

Breakfast:

Calories:

Lunch:

Calories:

Dinner:

Calories:

Snack:

Calories:

Water Intake

☐ **Vegetables&Fruits**
☐ **Meats&Seafood**
☐ **Eggs, Nuts& Seeds**
☐ **Healthy Oils**

Vitamins

Medicine

🏋 Today's Workout	CALORIES	WEIGHT

Today I feel.....

NOTES

Wake Time

Sleep Time

Paleo Food Log

Day 10

DATE:

JAN FEB MAR APR MAY JUN JUL AUG SEP OCT NOV DEC

Breakfast:

Calories:

Lunch:

Calories:

Dinner:

Calories:

Snack:

Calories:

Water Intake

Vitamins

Medicine

- [ ] Vegetables&Fruits
- [ ] Meats&Seafood
- [ ] Eggs, Nuts& Seeds
- [ ] Healthy Oils

Today's Workout	CALORIES	WEIGHT

Today I feel.....

NOTES

Wake Time

Sleep Time

Paleo Food Log

Day 11

DATE:

JAN FEB MAR APR MAY JUN JUL AUG SEP OCT NOV DEC

🍴 Breakfast:

Calories: _____

🍴 Lunch:

Calories: _____

🍴 Dinner:

Calories: _____

🍴 Snack:

Calories: _____

Water Intake

🥤🥤🥤🥤🥤🥤🥤🥤🥤🥤

☐ **Vegetables&Fruits**
☐ **Meats&Seafood**
☐ **Eggs, Nuts& Seeds**
☐ **Healthy Oils**

Vitamins [_____]   **Medicine** [_____]

🏋 Today's Workout	CALORIES	WEIGHT

Today I feel.....

😊 😠 😆
😓 😍 😋

NOTES

_____
_____
_____
_____

Wake Time (clock)

Paleo Food Log

Sleep Time (clock)

DATE:

JAN FEB MAR APR MAY JUN JUL AUG SEP OCT NOV DEC

Breakfast:

Calories:

Lunch:

Calories:

Dinner:

Calories:

Snack:

Calories:

Water Intake

☐ Vegetables&Fruits
☐ Meats&Seafood
☐ Eggs, Nuts& Seeds
☐ Healthy Oils

Vitamins [　　　　　]　Medicine [　　　　　]

🏋 Today's Workout	CALORIES	WEIGHT

Today I feel.....

NOTES

Wake Time

Sleep Time

Paleo Food Log

Day 13

DATE:

JAN FEB MAR APR MAY JUN JUL AUG SEP OCT NOV DEC

Breakfast:

Calories: _____

Lunch:

Calories: _____

Dinner:

Calories: _____

Snack:

Calories: _____

Water Intake

Vitamins [   ]   Medicine [   ]

☐ Vegetables&Fruits
☐ Meats&Seafood
☐ Eggs, Nuts& Seeds
☐ Healthy Oils

⫢ Today's Workout	CALORIES	WEIGHT

Today I feel.....

NOTES

_____
_____
_____
_____

Wake Time

Sleep Time

Paleo Food Log

Day 14

DATE:

JAN FEB MAR APR MAY JUN JUL AUG SEP OCT NOV DEC

Breakfast:

Calories:

Lunch:

Calories:

Dinner:

Calories:

Snack:

Calories:

Water Intake

Vitamins

Medicine

- [ ] Vegetables&Fruits
- [ ] Meats&Seafood
- [ ] Eggs, Nuts& Seeds
- [ ] Healthy Oils

Today's Workout	CALORIES	WEIGHT

Today I feel.....

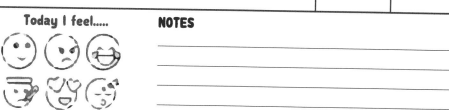

NOTES

Wake Time

Sleep Time

Paleo Food Log

Day 15

DATE:

JAN FEB MAR APR MAY JUN JUL AUG SEP OCT NOV DEC

Breakfast:

Calories: ....

Lunch:

Calories: ....

Dinner:

Calories: ....

Snack:

Calories: ....

Water Intake

☐ **Vegetables&Fruits**
☐ **Meats&Seafood**
☐ **Eggs, Nuts& Seeds**
☐ **Healthy Oils**

🖊 **Vitamins** [   ]   ● **Medicine** [   ]

🏋 Today's Workout	CALORIES	WEIGHT

Today I feel.....

NOTES
_____
_____
_____
_____

Wake Time

Sleep Time

Paleo Food Log

DATE:

JAN FEB MAR APR MAY JUN JUL AUG SEP OCT NOV DEC

Breakfast:

Calories:

Lunch:

Calories:

Dinner:

Calories:

Snack:

Calories:

Water Intake

[ ] **Vegetables&Fruits**
[ ] **Meats&Seafood**
[ ] **Eggs, Nuts& Seeds**
[ ] **Healthy Oils**

Vitamins

Medicine

🏋 Today's Workout	CALORIES	WEIGHT

Today I feel.....

NOTES

Wake Time

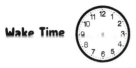 **Paleo Food Log**

Day 17

Sleep Time

DATE:

JAN FEB MAR APR MAY JUN JUL AUG SEP OCT NOV DEC

Breakfast:

Calories: ....

Lunch:

Calories: ....

Dinner:

Calories: ....

Snack:

Calories: ....

Water Intake

☐ **Vegetables&Fruits**
☐ **Meats&Seafood**
☐ **Eggs, Nuts& Seeds**
☐ **Healthy Oils**

Vitamins [   ]   Medicine [   ]

🏋 Today's Workout	CALORIES	WEIGHT

Today I feel.....

NOTES

_____
_____
_____
_____

Wake Time

Sleep Time

Paleo Food Log

DATE:

JAN FEB MAR APR MAY JUN JUL AUG SEP OCT NOV DEC

Breakfast:

Calories:

Lunch:

Calories:

Dinner:

Calories:

Snack:

Calories:

Water Intake

☐ Vegetables&Fruits
☐ Meats&Seafood
☐ Eggs, Nuts& Seeds
☐ Healthy Oils

Vitamins

Medicine

Today's Workout	CALORIES	WEIGHT

Today I feel.....

NOTES

Wake Time

Sleep Time

Paleo Food Log

Day 19

DATE:

JAN FEB MAR APR MAY JUN JUL AUG SEP OCT NOV DEC

Breakfast:

Calories:

Lunch:

Calories:

Dinner:

Calories:

Snack:

Calories:

Water Intake

☐ Vegetables&Fruits
☐ Meats&Seafood
☐ Eggs, Nuts& Seeds
☐ Healthy Oils

Vitamins _____

Medicine _____

🏋 Today's Workout	CALORIES	WEIGHT

Today I feel.....

NOTES

Wake Time

Sleep Time

Paleo Food Log

| Day 20 |

DATE:

JAN FEB MAR APR MAY JUN JUL AUG SEP OCT NOV DEC

Breakfast:

Calories:

Lunch:

Calories:

Dinner:

Calories:

Snack:

Calories:

Water Intake

☐ Vegetables&Fruits
☐ Meats&Seafood
☐ Eggs, Nuts& Seeds
☐ Healthy Oils

Vitamins

Medicine

🏋 Today's Workout	CALORIES	WEIGHT

Today I feel.....

NOTES

Wake Time

Sleep Time

Paleo Food Log

Day 21

DATE:

JAN FEB MAR APR MAY JUN JUL AUG SEP OCT NOV DEC

Breakfast:

Calories:

Lunch:

Calories:

Dinner:

Calories:

Snack:

Calories:

Water Intake

☐ Vegetables&Fruits
☐ Meats&Seafood
☐ Eggs, Nuts& Seeds
☐ Healthy Oils

Vitamins _____   Medicine _____

🏋 Today's Workout	CALORIES	WEIGHT

Today I feel.....

NOTES
_____
_____
_____
_____

Wake Time

Sleep Time

Paleo Food Log

Day 22

DATE:

Breakfast:

Calories:

Lunch:

Calories:

Dinner:

Calories:

Snack:

Calories:

Water Intake

☐ Vegetables&Fruits
☐ Meats&Seafood
☐ Eggs, Nuts& Seeds
☐ Healthy Oils

✎ Vitamins _____   ● Medicine _____

🏋 Today's Workout	CALORIES	WEIGHT

Today I feel.....

NOTES
_____
_____
_____
_____

Wake Time

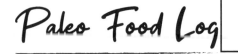 **Day 23**

DATE:

JAN FEB MAR APR MAY JUN JUL AUG SEP OCT NOV DEC

Sleep Time

Breakfast:

Calories: _____

Lunch:

Calories: _____

Dinner:

Calories: _____

Snack:

Calories: _____

Water Intake

Vitamins [   ]   **Medicine** [   ]

☐ Vegetables&Fruits
☐ Meats&Seafood
☐ Eggs, Nuts& Seeds
☐ Healthy Oils

🏋 Today's Workout	CALORIES	WEIGHT

Today I feel.....

NOTES

_____
_____
_____
_____

Paleo Food Log

Wake Time

Sleep Time

Day 24

DATE:

JAN FEB MAR APR MAY JUN JUL AUG SEP OCT NOV DEC

Breakfast:

Calories:

Lunch:

Calories:

Dinner:

Calories:

Snack:

Calories:

Water Intake

☐ Vegetables&Fruits
☐ Meats&Seafood
☐ Eggs, Nuts& Seeds
☐ Healthy Oils

Vitamins

Medicine

Today's Workout	CALORIES	WEIGHT

Today I feel.....

NOTES

Wake Time

Sleep Time

Paleo Food Log

| Day 25 |

DATE:

JAN FEB MAR APR MAY JUN JUL AUG SEP OCT NOV DEC

Breakfast:

Calories:

Lunch:

Calories:

Dinner:

Calories:

Snack:

Calories:

Water Intake

☐ **Vegetables&Fruits**
☐ **Meats&Seafood**
☐ **Eggs, Nuts& Seeds**
☐ **Healthy Oils**

Vitamins [ ]   **Medicine** [ ]

🏋 Today's Workout	CALORIES	WEIGHT

Today I feel.....

NOTES

Wake Time

Sleep Time

Paleo Food Log

Day 26

DATE:

JAN FEB MAR APR MAY JUN JUL AUG SEP OCT NOV DEC

Breakfast:

Calories:

Lunch:

Calories:

Dinner:

Calories:

Snack:

Calories:

Water Intake

Vitamins

Medicine

- [ ] Vegetables&Fruits
- [ ] Meats&Seafood
- [ ] Eggs, Nuts& Seeds
- [ ] Healthy Oils

Today's Workout	CALORIES	WEIGHT

Today I feel.....

NOTES

Wake Time

Sleep Time

Paleo Food Log

Day 27

DATE:

JAN FEB MAR APR MAY JUN JUL AUG SEP OCT NOV DEC

Breakfast:

Calories: _____

Lunch:

Calories: _____

Dinner:

Calories: _____

Snack:

Calories: _____

Water Intake

☐ Vegetables&Fruits
☐ Meats&Seafood
☐ Eggs, Nuts& Seeds
☐ Healthy Oils

Vitamins _____   Medicine _____

🏋 Today's Workout	CALORIES	WEIGHT

Today I feel.....

NOTES
_____
_____
_____
_____

Wake Time

Sleep Time

Paleo Food Log

DATE:

JAN FEB MAR APR MAY JUN JUL AUG SEP OCT NOV DEC

Breakfast:

Calories:

Lunch:

Calories:

Dinner:

Calories:

Snack:

Calories:

Water Intake

Vitamins

Medicine

☐ Vegetables&Fruits
☐ Meats&Seafood
☐ Eggs, Nuts& Seeds
☐ Healthy Oils

Today's Workout	CALORIES	WEIGHT

Today I feel.....

NOTES

Wake Time

Paleo Food Log

Day 20

DATE:

JAN FEB MAR APR MAY JUN JUL AUG SEP OCT NOV DEC

Sleep Time

Breakfast:

Calories: _____

Lunch:

Calories: _____

Dinner:

Calories: _____

Snack:

Calories: _____

Water Intake

☐ Vegetables&Fruits
☐ Meats&Seafood
☐ Eggs, Nuts& Seeds
☐ Healthy Oils

Vitamins [_____]   Medicine [_____]

🏋 Today's Workout	CALORIES	WEIGHT

Today I feel.....

NOTES
_____
_____
_____
_____

Wake Time

Sleep Time

Paleo Food Log

DATE:

JAN FEB MAR APR MAY JUN JUL AUG SEP OCT NOV DEC

Breakfast:

Calories:

Lunch:

Calories:

Dinner:

Calories:

Snack:

Calories:

Water Intake

- [ ] Vegetables&Fruits
- [ ] Meats&Seafood
- [ ] Eggs, Nuts& Seeds
- [ ] Healthy Oils

Vitamins

Medicine

🏋 Today's Workout	CALORIES	WEIGHT

Today I feel.....

NOTES

CONGRATS! YOU DID THAT ! YOU MADE IT!

Made in the USA
Columbia, SC
04 September 2023

22480139R00024